Living with Uveitis

A Complete Guide to Uveitis and Iritis

By Kevin Work

D1730344

By reading any document, the reader agrees that under no circumstances are we responsible for any losses, direct or indirect, which are incurred as a result of use of the information contained within this document, including – but not limited to errors, omissions, or inaccuracies.

Table of Contents

Introduction

The History of Uveitis

Understanding Autoimmune Diseases

What Is Uveitis and Iritis?

Testing for Uveitis and Iritis

Treatments for Uveitis and Iritis

Related Diseases

Uveitis and Diet

Iritis.org

Conclusion

Introduction

Finding out that you have a chronic disease – especially one with no known cure – can be deeply upsetting. We grow accustomed to our bodies doing what we want them to do when we want them to do it. A chronic disease upsets the status quo. Suddenly the things that we take for granted are no longer available to us.

These frustrations are compounded when the disease in question is one that is rare. It's bad enough to receive a diagnosis of a disease that is familiar. For example, diabetes is a chronic disease. It can be serious, but it is also something that most people understand. That doesn't mean that the diagnosis isn't upsetting, but people who are diagnosed with a known chronic disease have the comfort of knowing that their diagnosis is common. If they go home and look online to find information about diabetes, they will find thousands of websites containing helpful information. When they tell friends and family that they have diabetes, they don't have to explain what the disease is.

The same cannot be said of uveitis and iritis. While the basic explanation of the disease is simple, the fact remains that very few people who do not have uveitis know what it is. A person who is diagnosed with uveitis is likely to be met with blank stares and confusion when they share their diagnosis with friends and family. The confusion – and the need to explain – can make it harder to deal with an already-difficult situation.

Why I Decided to Write This Book

I was diagnosed with uveitis in 1994. That was in the days before the internet was widely used, and finding information about uveitis was difficult and frustrating. After I was diagnosed, I decided to start my own organization to provide information and support to other people who had uveitis and iritis.

My website, **Iritis.org**, is a place where people who have uveitis can turn to find detailed information about symptoms and treatments, as well as a large and supportive community of people who understand what it's like to live with uveitis. I started the organization with the hope that I could provide people with the support I couldn't find when I first got my diagnosis.

The reason I decided to write this book was to take the information that is available on my website and bring it all together into a single, easy-to-read book. While all of the information in the book is covered on my website and in the forums, it can be hard to piece together a complete picture of what it's like to have uveitis and what you can do to treat it. Some of the available information is highly technical and can be difficult for a layperson to understand. In this book, I'll use simple and straightforward language that will help you understand the complexities of uveitis.

The Rarity of Uveitis

As I stated before, one of the most frustrating things about having uveitis or iritis is that there is so little information available about the disease. It's not something most people know about. You might not expect your friends and family to be experts on a rare eye disease, but one of the things that surprised me in the beginning was how many doctors were unaware of uveitis. I was diagnosed with uveitis after having been misdiagnosed more than once, and it took ten years after my initial diagnosis to figure out that I had a related autoimmune disorder called ankylosing spondylitis as well.

The lack of knowledge in the medical community makes uveitis particularly challenging to diagnose and treat. Early diagnosis and immediate treatment are very important. If you don't get the treatments you need early, you can end up with serious complications. A misdiagnosis is not a minor thing, and with so many doctors being unaware of uveitis as a potential diagnosis, the potential for mistakes is high.

The goal of this book, then, is to provide you with detailed and straightforward information about what uveitis is, how it is treated, and other related issues.

What You Will Learn in This Book

The information in this book is designed to be a good introduction to uveitis and iritis for people who have just been diagnosed. In the first chapter, I'll give you a brief overview of the history of uveitis and iritis. While these diseases have been around for centuries, the names uveitis and iritis are relatively new. We'll talk about how ancient healers identified the symptoms associated with uveitis and iritis, and how treatment and diagnosis of the disease have evolved.

In the second chapter, I will go into detail explaining autoimmune diseases in general. The reason this is an important topic for people who have uveitis and iritis is that certain autoimmune disorders can be associated with uveitis. Autoimmune disorders are diseases that cause your immune system to attack parts of your body as if they were a threat. While some cases of uveitis have no identifiable cause, some (including mine) co-exist with autoimmune disorders.

The third chapter will explain what uveitis is, starting with a simple explanation of the biology of your eyes, and then explaining the different types of uveitis including iritis, pars planitis, chorioretinitis, and panuveitis. Most of us don't spend much time thinking about how our eyes work until we have a problem with them. I think it's important to start with the basics, so we'll begin with the eye and then move on to an explanation of the different types of uveitis as well as the symptoms associated with each.

In the fourth chapter, I'll cover the various tests and diagnostic tools that doctors use to diagnose uveitis. I'll talk about why it's so important to tell your doctor about every symptom you are experiencing, even the ones that do not appear to be related to your uveitis symptoms. I'll also talk about the importance of early and accurate diagnosis, and explain some of the most common complications associated with uveitis.

The fifth chapter will cover uveitis treatments, and why it is important to see a doctor and not attempt to treat the symptoms yourself. Typical over-the-counter treatments for inflamed eyes are not effective at treating uveitis. We'll cover anti-inflammatories including the various forms of corticosteroids: drops, oral medications, and implants. We'll also talk about some drugs that are used to suppress the immune system, thus cutting back on inflammation that may be the result of an overzealous immune response.

In the sixth chapter, we'll talk in detail about some of the diseases that can be linked with uveitis. Many people who have uveitis – even those who have been properly diagnosed – may find that they recognize some of the symptoms listed in this chapter. It is very important to make sure that you are getting treated for diseases and infections that can cause uveitis. The diseases covered will include autoimmune disorders, inflammatory disorders, viral infections, and bacterial infections.

After we have covered that, the next step is to talk about the effect that diet has on the inflammation that occurs in your body, and on your immune system. Uveitis is not a disease that can be managed with diet alone, but many people eat a diet that contains large amounts of foods that can cause or contribute to inflammation. For people who have chronic uveitis, eliminating inflammatory foods from their diets can help relieve symptoms and minimize the chances of repeated flare-ups of uveitis. I'll also talk about some foods that help to boost your immune system's performance, and some foods that specifically work to fight inflammation.

Finally, I'll tell you about the website for my organization. When I was first diagnosed, finding information about uveitis and iritis was very difficult. It was frustrating, and I decided to create a place where people who have uveitis can gather to learn, share their information, and provide support to one another. I'll give you an overview of the resources that are available there and a link so you can check it out for yourself.

By the time you are done reading this book, you will have comprehensive information about uveitis. You'll understand what causes it, what the symptoms are, and how it is treated. You'll also know what other diseases are linked to uveitis, and get some specific information about how you can modify your diet to help manage your symptoms.

Let's get started.

Chapter 1 – History of Uveitis

Uveitis is a relatively rare condition. Because of that, it can be easy to make the mistake of thinking that it's also a new disease – a perception that can be reinforced because so many doctors don't know about it.

The truth is that uveitis has been around for centuries.

Uveitis and Ancient Medicine

Since the discovery of antibiotics, modern medicine has made huge strides in understanding and treating diseases. People survive diseases today that would have had a high chance of killing them only a century ago, including things like tuberculosis and pneumonia.

Given that, why is there still so little understanding of uveitis? Why do patients who have it get misdiagnosed and shuffled around from doctor to doctor? There's clearly a fundamental lack of understanding about the disease, and yet it's not new.

Modern medicine is new, but human beings have practiced medicine for millennia. The ancient Egyptians, for example, had sophisticated medical knowledge. They documented the medical uses of thousands of herbs and plants and even performed rudimentary surgery.

The same is true for the Chinese. Chinese traditional medicine relies heavily on herbal treatments and the mind-body connection. The ancient Greeks, too, made great advances in medical knowledge. The Hippocratic Oath, which all physicians take today, is named after the legendary Greek doctor, Hippocrates.

Ancient Greek and Chinese doctors were very familiar with the symptoms of uveitis and iritis, as well as other diseases that we can clearly recognize today when we read their notes and observations. Of course, they didn't fully understand the causes of these diseases. They lacked the information we have about the immune system and inflammation, so their understanding was imperfect at best.

One of the most common misconceptions about uveitis amongst early doctors – and one that persisted into the 20th century – was that the disease occurred as the result of an infectious agent. The two most commonly named culprits were syphilis and tuberculosis, both of which were far more common in the past than they are today.

Over time, it became clear that no infection could account for all of the symptoms patients with uveitis experienced. As a result, doctors had to look for other explanations. In the 1960's and 1970's, the medical profession made huge strides in its work with antibodies, which started to point the way for people who were researching uveitis.

Today, the most up-to-date information available indicates that uveitis has no one single cause, but is due to the confluence of several different factors, including:

- Environmental factors

- Immunogenetics (a combination of genetic predisposition and reaction of the immune system)

- Endogenous dysregulation (a term indicating the fact that sometimes it's not possible to identify what causes uveitis)

The medical profession is still learning about the causes of uveitis, which is one of the things that can make having it so frustrating for patients. A quick review of online forums discussing uveitis reveals dozens of stories from patients who were repeatedly misdiagnosed.

Lack of Knowledge

Researchers in the field of ophthalmology are making uveitis research a priority, but there are still significant gaps in our understanding of what causes the disease. About two years ago, researchers at Mahajan Laboratories in Iowa City discovered that a mutation in a particular gene – the CAPN5 gene – may be responsible for the genetic disposition for uveitis. That knowledge is certainly important, but there is still a lot of work to be done to fill in the gaps and discover a cure.

Uveitis is considered a rare disease, which in the United States means that it affects between 20,000 and 200,000 people each year. The rarity of the disease means that it gets a lot less attention than some other disease. For example, breast cancer is fairly common and it gets a lot of attention – and research money. An entire month is dedicated to Breast Cancer Awareness every year, and screening is very common.

Contrast that with uveitis. If you don't have uveitis or know someone personally who has it, chances are you have never heard of it. Many doctors are unfamiliar with it as well. Because of its rarity, the experience of having uveitis can be extremely frustrating. Because of its link to the function of the immune system, uveitis often goes hand-in-hand with other diagnoses. Patients might be seeing their primary care physician for treatment of other issues and not connect the symptoms of uveitis with their other symptoms.

One of the key ways to overcome the lack of knowledge about uveitis and iritis is to talk about it. Understanding the disease's origins and history is the first step in that process. The next step is discussing autoimmune diseases in general before we get into the specifics of what uveitis is and how it affects the people who have it. In the next chapter, we'll do exactly that. I'll tell you how autoimmune disorders affect your body as a prelude to going into greater depth about uveitis and iritis.

Chapter 2 – Understanding Autoimmune Diseases

As I said in the introduction, uveitis is a disease that can go hand-in-hand with a whole class of diseases known as *autoimmune disorders*. What that means is that your immune system is attacking your body (in the case of uveitis, your eye) as if it were a harmful intruder. To understand fully what uveitis is, it's important to start by understanding autoimmune diseases in general – and that means taking a quick look at the immune system.

How Does the Immune System Work?

The human immune system is remarkably complex. It's composed of various cells and organs that all work together to protect your body from harm. For example, your immune system is what helps wounds to heal and helps prevent you from catching viruses. When any harmful agent – called an *antigen* – enters the human body, your immune system reacts.

Your immune system's reaction can vary depending on whether it recognizes the antigen or not. For example, if you had the chicken pox as a child and were exposed to the disease again as an adult, you most likely wouldn't catch it again. That's because when you have a virus, your body produces *antibodies* – specialized proteins that attack specific antigens. Once your body produces antibodies, you become immune to the antigen that they fight.

Leukocytes are cells that form an important part of your immune system. There are two basic types:

- Phagocytes are cells that attack invading antigens.

- Lymphocytes are specialized cells that remember antigens and help destroy them if you're exposed to them again.

There are various types of each cell. For example, *neutrophils* are a type of phagocyte that fight bacteria. One way that doctors can test for a bacterial infection is to measure the number of neutrophils in your blood.

There are two main types of lymphocytes, both of which are manufactured in your bone marrow. *B lymphocytes* locate antigens, produce antibodies, and send them to "tag" the virus or bacteria in question. *T lymphocytes* (also known as T cells) are the body's attack system. They seek out the cells that have been tagged with antibodies and destroy them.

There are three basic types of immunity:

- Innate immunity is the immunity that we're all born having. For example, there are certain diseases that animals get that don't affect humans. We are born with immunity to those diseases.

- Adaptive immunity is the kind of immunity we acquire throughout our lives. Older people, having been exposed to more antigens, tend to catch fewer viruses than children because their adaptive immunity is stronger than it is in children.

- Passive immunity is immunity that's borrowed from another source. One example is breastfeeding: nursing infants get temporary immunity because their mothers' breast milk contains antibodies.

Immunizations work by introducing antigens to the body in a way that doesn't cause sickness. The immunization forces the body to create antibodies that will attack the disease in the event you are exposed to it.

Immune Disorders

Like any other part of the human body, the immune system is not perfect. Sometimes it malfunctions. Let's look at a couple of quick examples:

- Allergies occur when your immune system overreacts to an antigen such as pollen, dust, or mold – which in this context is called *allergens*. Seasonal allergies are the most common type of allergy, but allergic disorders such as asthma and eczema are fairly common as well.

- Immunodeficiencies are diseases that can be either primary (meaning that a person is born with them) or acquired (meaning that you catch a disease that compromises your immune system). Examples of primary immunodeficiencies include Severe Combined Immunodeficiency (SCID), also known as the Bubble Boy disease, and DiGeorge Syndrome. Acquired immunodeficiencies include HIV and immunodeficiencies caused by medications such as those used in chemotherapy.

The third type of immunodeficiency is the autoimmune disorder.

What Are Autoimmune Disorders?

Building on the foundation of what we just learned about the immune system, now it's time to talk briefly about autoimmune disorders. An autoimmune disorder is a disease that causes your body's immune system to attack parts of your body as if they were antigens. For example, rheumatoid arthritis is an autoimmune disorder that causes the body to attack connective tissues, including ligaments, joints, and tendons, as though they were harmful to the body.

One way to look at these disorders is to view them as a misfiring of the immune system. Under ideal conditions, the immune system would only attack things that were truly harmful. Sometimes, though, the system gets confused; and when that happens, it can attack healthy cells as though they were harmful.

The frustrating thing about autoimmune disorders in general – and uveitis in particular – is that it is unclear what causes the body to turn on itself in this way. There are several theories. One is that there might be a genetic component, something that makes certain people more likely to develop autoimmune disorders than other people. Another theory is that certain viruses, bacteria, and drugs may trigger autoimmune reactions.

Symptoms of autoimmune disorders can vary widely from disease to disease, but some of the most common symptoms are fatigue and a feeling of general malaise.

Treatments for autoimmune diseases usually focus on two primary things:

1. Offering relief from the symptoms associated with the disease

2. Maintaining your body's ability to fight disease and infection

Both are important. When you have an autoimmune disorder, you don't want to suppress your immune system. You still need it to protect you from antigens. In some cases, such as Celiac disease (an autoimmune disorder that's related to gluten consumption) the symptoms can be controlled by eliminating certain foods from your diet. Many people with autoimmune disorders cut inflammatory foods out of their diet – something we'll talk about in greater detail later in the book.

Now that you have a general understanding of what an autoimmune disorder is, the next step is to talk about uveitis in particular – and that's what we'll cover in the next chapter.

Chapter 3 – What Is Uveitis and Iritis

One of the most frustrating things about getting a diagnosis of uveitis is realizing how little information is available about the disease. Human beings have a natural curiosity about life in general; and when we're sick, our inclination is to research and learn so we can do a better job of advocating for ourselves.

Simply put, uveitis is an inflammation of the part of the eye known as the uvea. That makes it sound very simple – and in some ways it is. But the goal of this book is not to give you the simple explanation. It's to give you as much information as possible so you have a full understanding of what's happening to your body, and why. With that in mind, this chapter will talk in detail about iritis and uveitis (as well as some less common forms of the disease), starting with an explanation of the biology of your eyes.

How the Eyes Work

Perhaps the simplest way to start to explain how human eyes work is to say that they are a bit like cameras. When you take a photograph, you look through the camera's viewfinder. You adjust the focus to make sure the picture you take is clear and defined. Depending on the available lighting, you might choose to use a flash to make the image easier to see. You might also move to a different location or shift your perspective in order to get a better image. Your eyes work in a similar way.

The *cornea* is a transparent organ at the front of your eye that receives the light your eyes take in, similar to the manner in which a camera lens focuses an image. All eyesight starts with light, which gets reflected by the objects we see. While some parts of our body can be seriously injured and still be functional, the cornea cannot. It's very sensitive, and even a small injury can cause significant problems with your vision.

After reflected light passes through the cornea, it encounters the *crystalline lens*, which sits directly behind the pupil. As the name suggests, the crystalline lens is transparent. It is filled with a colorless liquid called *aqueous humor*. The eyes' lenses are held in place by a ring of muscles called *ciliary muscles*. In addition to holding the lenses in place, the ciliary muscles also help the lenses to make adjustments. For example, when you try to see an object that's far away, the muscles relax, causing the lenses to flatten so you can see farther. By contrast, when you're trying to see something that's close to you, the muscles contract, and the lenses thicken.

After your lenses focus the light, it gets sent to the *iris*. The iris is a ring-shaped, pigmented membrane. It's the part of your eye that determines your eye color. At the center of the iris is the *pupil*, which is the black circle in the middle of your eye. When light passes through the pupil, it can make the pupil *dilate* (become larger) or *constrict* (become smaller.) If you are in very bright light, your pupils typically constrict, and when you are in dim light, they dilate to help you see better.

Behind the iris is the rest of your eyeball, which is filled with a jelly-like substance called *vitreous humor*. This part of the eye also contains the blood vessels that that get rid of waste products and supply your eyes with the nutrients they need to work properly. The light that enters through your pupil and the iris must pass through the vitreous humor before it reaches your *retina*.

The retina is the nerve center of the eye. It contains two different types of nerve receptors called *rods* and *cones*. The rods process monochrome visual signals in low light while the cones detect colors and fine details. There are three different kinds of cones: red absorbing, green absorbing, and blue absorbing. Your brain interprets colors by evaluating the relative activity of the three different kinds of cones. The cones are located in a section of the eye called the *fovea*, which is responsible for the sharpness of your vision. When the light received by your eyes strikes either the rods or cones in your retina, it is converted into an electric impulse that is then transmitted to your brain via the *optic nerve*.

One of the things that make human vision unique in the animal kingdom is that it is *binocular,* meaning that we see the images received by both eyes as a single picture. This is possible because the optic nerves from each eye intersect and transmit some of their signals to the opposite side of the brain over something called the *optic chiasm* in a process called *decussation.* Decussation allows your brain to fuse the two images into one cohesive image. Without this ability, you might wind up with two slightly different pictures as a result of looking with both eyes. It's also interesting to note that the images from your left eye go to the right side of your brain and vice versa.

Once your brain receives the electrical impulses from the optic nerve, part of what it does is to compress the data. The reason that happens is that there are about 125 million receptor cells in the retina, but only about one million *axons* (nerve fibers) in the optic nerve. That means that a 125 to 1 reduction of data needs to take place for the axons to receive accurate visual information from the retina.

Another interesting thing about the way your brain processes images is that it does it in stages. First, it receives lines and edges – the general outline of things. Next, it gets movement, form and color, and then it puts everything together to create a detailed image. The information travels through your optic nerves to a part of the brain called the *thalamus* – more specifically, to the *lateral geniculate nucleus* (LGN). The LGN works like a relay station for visual impulses. It sends signals to the *primary visual cortex* using a process known as optic radiation. The primary visual cortex is located at the back of the brain in an area called the *occipital cortex*. You also have a *secondary visual cortex* that's responsible for processing more complex visual signals.

From the visual cortices, the information is transmitted to various parts of the brain. The *ventral pathway* leads to the temporal lobe, where memory is stored, and it is primarily used to help you recognize objects. The *dorsal pathway* leads to the parietal lobe, and it is used to help you locate objects.

As you can see, human eyes are both complex and remarkably sensitive. Now that you understand how they work let's talk about how uveitis affects them.

What Is Uveitis?

Uveitis is often used as a catch-all term for inflammation of the middle part of your eye, called the uvea. There are several types of uveitis that can be defined by the part of the uvea affected. Anterior uveitis is the most common, but let's look quickly at each type.

Anterior Uveitis

Anterior uveitis, which can also be called *iritis* or *iridocyclitis*, is an inflammation of the iris and the *anterior chamber* – the fluid-filled part of the eye between the cornea and the retina. Iridocyclitis is a variation of uveitis that is typified by inflammation of the *ciliary chamber* – the area where the ciliary muscles are located.

As stated previously, anterior uveitis is the most common form of uveitis, accounting for approximately two-thirds to 90% of all diagnosed cases. Anterior uveitis may be either acute (occurring one time) or chronic (recurring many times.) The symptoms of anterior uveitis include:

- Redness of the eyes
- Blurred vision
- Eye pain
- Photophobia (sensitivity to light)
- Headaches
- Floaters (dark spots that appear in your field of vision)

Signs that can help an ophthalmologist or doctor to diagnose anterior uveitis include:

- *Keratic precipitates* (inflammatory deposits) on the surface of the cornea

- *Hypopeon* (inflammatory cells) in the anterior chamber

- Dilated ciliary vessels

- *Busacca nodules* (inflammatory nodules) on the surface of the iris, most common in particular forms of anterior uveitis including Fuchs' heterochromic iridocyclitis

- *Synechia* (a condition in which the iris adheres to either the cornea or the lens)

When anterior uveitis is acute, it will typically respond to treatment and not return. When it is chronic, treatments do not prevent it from returning.

Intermediate Uveitis

Like anterior uveitis, intermediate uveitis involves inflammation of the uvea. What makes it different is that the inflammation involves the cells in the vitreous cavity instead of the iris. This form of the disease is also known as *pars planitis*. The *pars plana* is part of the ciliary body. Here are the most common symptoms of intermediate uveitis:

- Floaters
- Blurred vision
- Pain
- Photophobia

This type of uveitis generally occurs in only one eye at a time. Some of the signs that can help doctors diagnose intermediate uveitis include:

- *Snowbanking* – the deposit of inflammatory particles on the pars plana

- *Snowballs* – inflammatory cells that form in the vitreous humor

Intermediate uveitis is less common than anterior uveitis.

Posterior Uveitis

Posterior uveitis is an inflammation of the posterior (rear) part of the uvea, including the retina and *choroid* (the area of the uvea behind the retina). This form of uveitis is also sometimes called *chorioretinitis*. The most common symptoms include:

- Blurred vision
- Floaters
- Pain or redness in the eyes
- Excessive tearing
- *Photopsia* (seeing flashing lights)

When inflammation occurs in the choroid but not the retina, it is called *choroiditis*.

Pan-uveitis

As you might suspect from the name, pan-uveitis is an inflammation of all parts of the uvea, including the iris, choroid, and the ciliary body.

Causes of Uveitis

One of the first things people want to know when they are diagnosed with a disease is what caused them to get sick in the first place. With a diagnosis of uveitis, the answer to that question can be difficult – or even impossible – to determine. There are multiple things that can cause inflammation of the uvea, and sometimes it occurs for no apparent reason. In fact, in about 50% of the diagnosed uveitis cases, the disease is listed as *idiopathic*, which means that the diagnosing physician has not been able to determine what caused the patient to become ill.

In the other 50% of cases, there is a determining cause. In this section, we will talk about some of the most common causes of uveitis.

Eye Trauma or Surgery

Trauma and surgery are both potential causes of inflammation in any part of the body. Inflammation is part of your immune system's natural response to injury or infection, so it stands to reason that if your eye is injured, whether in an accident or during surgery, the eye could become inflamed as a result. In any patient who presents with uveitis after surgery, the diagnosing physician should consider the surgery as a potential cause of the inflammation.

Bacterial or Viral Infections

As stated above, inflammation is caused by your body fighting antigens including viruses and bacteria. If you become exposed to certain infectious agents, the inflammation can spread to one or both eyes. Remember that in the past, uveitis was linked specifically to two infectious diseases: tuberculosis, and syphilis.

Other infections that have been linked to uveitis include:

- Herpes simplex virus
- Lyme disease
- Infectious hepatitis
- Leprosy
- West Nile virus
- Human immunodeficiency virus (HIV)
- Toxoplasmosis (bacterial infection)
- Histoplasmosis (fungal infection)
- Viral meningitis

In addition, uveitis may occur if the eye comes into direct contact with a toxic substance such as a poison or chemical.

Autoimmune Disorders

You already know that uveitis is linked to certain autoimmune and inflammatory disorders that affect other parts of your body. Later in the book I'll talk in depth about some of the diseases that most often coexist with uveitis, but for now let's just list them:

- Ankylosing spondylitis
- Arthritis
- Behcet's syndrome
- Crohn's disease
- Kawasaki disease
- Lupus erythematosus
- Psoriasis
- Rheumatoid arthritis
- Sarcoidosis
- Ulcerative colitis

One of the things that make diagnosing uveitis so difficult is that it may be one of many symptoms that patients experience. For example, a patient with rheumatoid arthritis would experience pain and swelling in the joints and difficulty moving as well as inflammation in the eyes. An ophthalmologist who had experience with uveitis might recognize the symptoms, but a general practitioner might not.

What Is It Like to Live with Uveitis?

Talking about the symptoms of uveitis is a good place to start, but symptoms paint an incomplete picture of what it's like to live with a chronic disease in general, or with uveitis in particular. Most people hear a term like "eye pain," and they think that it's like having a headache – unpleasant, but not debilitating. In this section, we'll talk about some of the difficulties that people with chronic uveitis face.

Inability to Drive

People who have relatively mild attacks of uveitis can still drive; but for people who experience severe inflammation, it can be impossible. Photosensitivity can make it very difficult to see, and the eye pain and related symptoms can be debilitating. Some people experience temporary vision loss when they have a flare-up of uveitis, and that makes it impossible for them to drive. Blurred vision and floaters are some of the most common symptoms of uveitis, and it is unsafe to drive when you can't see properly.

Uveitis patients who rely on their cars to get to and from work or school may find that their lives are totally disrupted by a serious episode of uveitis. It's not uncommon for people to need to visit the doctor on a near-daily basis to monitor the inflammation. If they are unable to drive themselves, they need to rely on someone else to take them where they need to go.

Lost Work and Wages

Related to the inability to drive is the fact that many people with serious, chronic uveitis find that they are unable to work during a flare-up. Transportation to and from work may be part of the problem, but impaired vision can also make it difficult to perform many jobs. For example, a teacher who needs to grade student tests and papers may be unable to see to do her work. The same is true of a nurse who needs to see patient charts and read dosages on containers of medicines.

Many employers have rules about how much work an employee can miss and still keep his/her job. It is not uncommon for people who have chronic uveitis to end up losing their jobs or having other difficulties as a result of the disease.

Vision Loss

Floaters and blurry vision are common symptoms of uveitis, and when people experience flare-ups that last for a long time, they can experience serious and debilitating vision loss. The lack of information about uveitis sometimes leads to treatments that can help in the short term but don't provide long-term solutions. For example, a person who experienced serious vision loss might have surgery to remove deposits in the vitreous humor. However, in the absence of a comprehensive, long-term treatment plan, the deposits can build up again over time.

Frustration and Depression

For a lot of people, their self-esteem and feelings of usefulness are directly tied to their ability to work and function. People who have chronic uveitis may find that they are unable to work, and that can lead to frustration, anxiety, and depression. Feelings of frustration are very common because many doctors are not aware of the best way to treat uveitis and may be dismissive of patients' symptoms and difficulties. It is fairly common for patients with uveitis to be misdiagnosed at first, as the symptoms are easily confused with those of conjunctivitis or allergies.

Another thing that can contribute to patient frustration is the fact that often there is no way to determine what has caused a uveitis flare-up. As stated previously, sometimes uveitis is co-diagnosed with autoimmune disorders such as ankylosing spondylitis. However, sometimes repeated testing reveals no definitive cause.

Some patients find that using steroid drops –
something we'll talk more about later in the book –
can help. However, some people find that as soon as
they stop using the drops, the inflammation returns.

The fact is that chronic uveitis is extremely
frustrating and debilitating to live with in the long
term. The combination of pain and discomfort, vision
problems, loss of mobility, and the inability to work
can all add up to an experience that's hugely
upsetting to the people who have it. It doesn't help
that most people who haven't experienced it don't
know about uveitis. It's not a common disease, and
the lack of knowledge about it can be frustrating for
patients as well.

In the next chapter, we'll talk about the tests that
doctors use to determine if a patient has uveitis.

Chapter 4 – Testing for Uveitis and Iritis

Now that we have discussed the symptoms and causes of uveitis, it's time to talk in detail about how your doctor or ophthalmologist can diagnose uveitis. Many of us turn to over the counter medications as our first line of defense when we get sick. However, using regular eye drops will not help to ease the symptoms of uveitis. Patients typically end up visiting their doctors fairly soon after symptoms first appear because the medicines they can get without a prescription are not effective.

It is important for patients who have uveitis to share all symptoms with their doctors even if they appear to be unrelated to uveitis. As we discussed in the previous chapter, uveitis often occurs as a result of another disease, most typically an autoimmune or inflammatory disorder. When you share all of your existing symptoms with your doctor, you have the best chance of receiving an accurate diagnosis.

Medical History

The first thing any doctor should do when they see a patient is to take a full medical history. If you are referred to a specialist by your primary care doctor, you should be prepared to answer questions about your medical history and other symptoms. A full medical history is an essential diagnostic tool because it can help to identify underlying diseases or infections that may be causing or contributing to uveitis.

From the patient's perspective, it's important to note all symptoms you are having. You may think that your digestive problems have nothing to do with the inflammation in your eyes, but that's not necessarily true. One of the frustrating things about modern medical treatment is that in some situations, patients only get a few minutes with the doctor, and the tendency may be to treat symptoms without investigating their root cause. Patients can increase the chances of getting proper treatment by listing every symptom.

Physical Examination

After a complete medical history is taken, the next step in diagnosing uveitis and iritis is to do a physical examination of the eyes. There are several clear markers that indicate a diagnosis of uveitis, including:

- Anterior chamber flare. Anterior chamber flare is a condition that occurs when there is a severe inflammation of the blood vessels in the eyes. When that happens, protein can leak from the vessels into the aqueous humor and make it appear cloudy instead of clear. A doctor can spot anterior chamber flare by shining a thin beam of light into the eye and watching to see if the beam of light is dispersed by the cloudiness – hence the term *flare*. This is a classic sign of inflammation.

- Synechiae. Synechiae are adhesions (abnormal fusions that bind two tissues together) that occur in cases of severe inflammation. Patients with uveitis may experience synechiae binding the iris to the cornea, a condition called anterior synechiae. Alternatively, the iris may become bound to the lens, a condition that is called posterior synechiae.

- Keratic precipitates. Keratic precipitates are inflamed cells that accumulate in the anterior part of the cornea, which is also known as the endothelial area. When the cells clump together, they form white spots that are visible upon inspection. When the keratic precipitates appear large and greasy or granular, the patient has granulatamous uveitis. Generally this type of uveitis is associated with an underlying cause of tuberculosis or sarcoidosis.

- Retinal lesions. Retinal lesions are sores that appear on the retina. While less common than the other physical signs of uveitis listed, retinal lesions may point to underlying conditions such as retinal tumors.

- HLA-B27 Gene. The Human Leukocyte Antigen gene is responsible for providing instructions for making a protein that is involved in the body's immune system. The B27 is a marker for a certain protein that decides what are healthy cells and what are foreign invaders inside the body. A blood test can be performed to check for the HLA-B27 marker. A positive test means the HLA-B27 gene is present and increases your chance of autoimmune disorders. This gene is strongly associated with arthritis conditions such as ankylosing spondylitis.

In addition to the signs listed above, here are some other signs your doctor may look for to determine whether you have uveitis.

Physical signs of anterior uveitis may include:

- Reduced visual acuity (clearness) in the affected eye

- The pupil in the affected eye may be a different size or shape than the pupil in the unaffected eye

- Direct photophobia (shining a light into the affected eye) or consensual photophobia (shining a light into the unaffected eye)

- Redness and inflammation of the conjunctiva (the thin skin inside the eyelids and around the eyes)

- The most characteristic sign of anterior uveitis is the presence of particles in the aqueous humor. The particles can be seen by shining a light into the eye, and may appear similar to motes of dust floating in a ray of light.

The main physical signs of intermediate uveitis include:

- Inflammatory cells in the vitreous humor

- Snowbanking or snowballs (large particles as discussed previously)

Finally, the most common visual signs of posterior uveitis include:

- Retinal lesions

- Inflammation of the retinal veins (retinal vasculitis)

- Edema (swelling) of the optic nerve

Once the physical examination has been completed, there may be a need for additional diagnostic tests. With anterior uveitis, additional testing may not be necessary unless it is to help determine underlying causes. However, when the uveitis is in the posterior section of the uvea, it may be necessary to use imaging techniques to get a clear picture of the problem. Some of the tests that may be used are:

- Fundus fluorescein angiography. This is a diagnostic test that uses dye to allow your doctor to see the back of your eye more clearly. In the test, a dye is typically injected into the patient's arm. The dye travels to the eye where it highlights the blood vessels. Your doctor will then take photographs that will enable him to see inflammation or leakage in the blood vessels.

- Optical coherence tomography. This is a non-invasive diagnostic test that uses light waves to scan your eye and measure the thickness of the retina. It can be used as a tool to help measure retinal damage. In addition to helping diagnose uveitis, it can also be used to pinpoint damage to the eyes from diabetes complications, macular edema, age-related macular degeneration, and retinopathy.

Laboratory Tests

It is rare for laboratory testing to be required for uveitis, but in situations where the diagnosis is difficult to make, or the doctor suspects an infectious agent or malignancy may be causing the inflammation, he/she may want to take a sample of the aqueous humor. This procedure is done using a thin needle and typical local or general anesthetic.

It is rare for uveitis to be properly diagnosed by a general practitioner. Even in cases where it is diagnosed by an ophthalmologist, the usual procedure would be to immediately refer the patient to a specialist to confirm the diagnosis and begin treatment.

Treatment of uveitis is often a complicated affair. Treating the symptoms of uveitis is relatively straightforward; but because uveitis is often complicated by other diseases, the treatments must take those into account, too.

Importance of Early Treatment

One of the things that it is important for people who have uveitis to understand is that it is essential to get an accurate diagnosis and immediate treatment. There are some diseases that people can live with for long periods of time without running into serious problems, but uveitis and iritis are not among them.

The problem with leaving uveitis untreated – or insufficiently treated – is that prolonged inflammation can lead to serious complications. Let's talk about some of the potential complications associated with untreated uveitis.

Glaucoma

Glaucoma is a very serious eye disease caused by the buildup of pressure on the optic nerve. It can be hereditary, but it can also be caused by inflammatory diseases such as uveitis and iritis. What happens is that pressure builds up in the aqueous humor, and it applies stress to the optic nerve. If it's left untreated, glaucoma can lead to permanent vision loss and even blindness.

Glaucoma is not common in patients who have uveitis, but it is important to be aware that if you feel pressure in your eyes, you should tell your doctor. The longer pressure is applied to the optic nerve, the more serious the damage can become.

One reason it is so important to be aware of the risk of glaucoma is that patients who take corticosteroids such as prednisone are more susceptible to the disease than patients who don't. Since corticosteroids are the most common treatment for uveitis, you need to know that the risk exists so you can let your doctor know if you experience any of the warning signs of glaucoma.

Cataracts

Simply put, a cataract is a cloudiness in the lenses of your eyes. Some cataracts are very small and may not even be noticeable to the person who has them while others can be large and may require surgery.

The most common symptoms of cataracts are cloudy or blurred vision, difficulty seeing at night due to the glare from lights, glare from lamps or the sun, and double vision. If you experience any of these symptoms or notice any cloudiness in your eyes, you should see a doctor immediately.

Cataracts are more likely to develop in people who have chronic uveitis because, like glaucoma, long-term use of corticosteroids is a risk factor. There are other factors that may affect the probability that you will develop cataracts, including heredity, age, and whether or not you smoke.

Retinal Detachment

Another potential complication of untreated uveitis is *retinal detachment*. As we discussed earlier, the retina is the part of the eye that interprets light and color. It is located at the back of the uvea and can become inflamed in patients with posterior uveitis.

Retinal detachment occurs when the retina becomes detached from the tissue that surrounds it. It is a very serious condition that requires immediate treatment by a doctor. The most common symptoms include seeing flashing lights, the sudden appearance of floaters, and darkening of your peripheral (side) vision. Retinal detachment does not hurt, so these symptoms are the only warning signs that detachment has occurred. Sometimes people may experience a retinal tear first, which is characterized by some of the same symptoms. Anytime you experience new vision problems such as floaters or flashing lights, you should see your eye doctor.

It is very important to treat retinal attachment. If it is left untreated, you can experience permanent vision loss.

Optic Nerve Damage

The final complication associated with untreated uveitis is damage to the optic nerve. Glaucoma also damages the optic nerve, but you don't have to have glaucoma to experience nerve damage. The reason it is so important to keep your optic nerve healthy is that your nerves have only a limited ability to repair themselves and regenerate. If your optic nerve is damaged, it can result in permanent vision loss.

As you can see, getting immediate and ongoing treatment for uveitis is extremely important. Not only is untreated uveitis uncomfortable, but it can also lead to very serious consequences including permanent loss of vision.

In the next chapter, we will talk about the most common treatments for uveitis, including dosages, effectiveness, and potential side effects.

Chapter 5 – Treatments for Uveitis and Iritis

Once a patient has been diagnosed with uveitis, the next step is to come up with a course of treatment. Depending on the location of the uveitis, treatments may vary. Typically, the treatments focus on accomplishing the following things:

1. Reducing inflammation
2. Relieving eye pain
3. Improving vision and restoring vision loss
4. Prevent tissue damage

As stated in the previous chapter, the treatments for uveitis must go hand in hand with treatments for any underlying causes or diseases. Let's start with the most common treatments for anterior uveitis, and then we'll talk about some of the treatments for uveitis in other areas of the eye.

Corticosteroid Drops

By far the most common treatment for anterior uveitis is a prescription of eye drops containing corticosteroids. Although steroids are often associated with improved athletic performance, their primary function is as a powerful anti-inflammatory.

Corticosteroids work by mimicking the effects of hormones that your body's adrenal glands – which sit on top of the kidneys – produce naturally. Having a higher-than-normal level of these hormones, as you do when you take corticosteroids, reduces inflammation. It also acts as a natural suppressant for the immune system, something that can be helpful for patients with autoimmune disorders.

Some of the corticosteroids that are used in eye drops include:

- Prednisone
- Hydrocortisone
- Loteprednol

- Dexamethasone

When steroids are used topically, side effects can occur including irritation, itching, swelling, and redness. In some cases, they can also cause pressure to build up in the eye. It is important to see your doctor regularly if you are using any type of steroid medication.

Oral or Injected Corticosteroids

Eye drops with corticosteroids are usually the first treatment your doctor will try if you have uveitis, but eye drops are not always effective. If that happens, your doctor will most likely switch you to an oral corticosteroid medication.

Taking oral corticosteroids affects your entire body. They work in the same way, but because you are ingesting them the risk of side effects is higher than it would be with a topical steroid. Some of the most common side effects associated with taking oral steroids include:

- Fluid retention
- Increased pressure in the eyes (glaucoma)
- Increased blood pressure
- Weight gain
- Mood swings

Taking oral steroids for a long period of time, as some patients with chronic uveitis must do, carries a risk for additional side effects including increased blood sugar, increased risk of infections, cataracts, osteoporosis (thinning bones), decreased hormone production, slower healing of wounds, and susceptibility to bruises.

Another option is for your doctor to inject corticosteroids into the affected eye. Because there are some risks associated with the injections, most doctors will only do this procedure three or four times a year at most. The side effects of injected corticosteroids include:

- Infection

- Pain
- Shrinking of soft tissue at the injection site
- Fading of skin (loss of pigmentation)

Immunosuppressive Medications

When uveitis is caused or exacerbated by an autoimmune disorder, or when a patient doesn't respond to corticosteroids, a doctor will sometimes prescribe medications that help to suppress the immune system. While normally suppressing the immune system isn't a good thing, when a patient has an autoimmune disorder it may be necessary to help manage the disease. Some of the most commonly prescribed medications include:

- Methotrexate
- Mycophenolate
- Azathioprine
- Cyclosporine

Implantations

People who have posterior uveitis, which is not treatable with eye drops, may respond well to a new treatment that involves transplanting a time-release capsule into the eye. The capsule releases corticosteroid medication slowly. Overall, patients who had the implant responded more quickly than patients who took oral corticosteroids; but they also have an increased chance of serious side effects such as glaucoma and cataracts.

Biologics

One of the most promising new treatments for uveitis is the use of biologics. Biologics are drugs that were originally developed to treat systemic inflammatory diseases such as lupus, and to protect people who had received organ transplants. Testing of these drugs to treat uveitis and iritis is still in its early stages, but the early results are promising.

Simply put, biologics are natural proteins that work with the body to suppress inflammatory reactions. They contain proteins that work to block particular functions of the immune system, including those that may lead to atypical autoimmune responses. These drugs have been approved as treatments for certain autoimmune disorders, but they are not yet approved for use in the treatment of ocular inflammation.

Surgeries

Surgery is usually a last resort for treating uveitis and is used only in cases where the patient is not responding to corticosteroids and the doctor fears that there may be permanent damage to the eyes. Technically, the implantation process described above is a surgery. The other surgery that is sometimes performed on people with uveitis is called *vitrectomy*.

Vitrectomy is a surgery that is performed to remove vitreous humor from the eye. It may be done when the humor becomes cloudy due to blood leakage. It is also sometimes necessary in the case of retinal detachment or other problems with the retina because removing the humor can help a doctor get to the retina more easily.

Having a vitrectomy can help restore vision when a patient has experienced severe hemorrhaging in the eyes. Any surgery carries the risk of complications and side effects. Some of the potential side effects of vitrectomy are decreased vision, increased pain, fluid build-up in the eye, redness, swelling, infection, and cataracts.

Treatment with corticosteroids is by far the most common treatment for uveitis. Patients who take steroids long term must be monitored by a physician to make sure that potentially-serious complications are caught early.

As I mentioned earlier, about half of all uveitis cases are idiopathic, meaning that a doctor is not able to pinpoint an underlying cause for the disease.

However, the other 50% of cases are linked to an underlying cause. There are several types of diseases that commonly coexist with uveitis, including autoimmune disorders, inflammatory disorders, and certain infectious diseases. We'll talk about some of the most common ones in the next chapter.

Chapter 6 – Related Diseases

One of the things that makes treating uveitis so tricky is the fact that it often occurs as a result of another disease. What that means in practical terms is that it can be difficult for doctors to diagnose uveitis because other symptoms may confuse things. In this chapter, we'll talk about some of the diseases that are most likely to coexist with uveitis. This information can be helpful for patients who may not be aware that other symptoms they are experiencing are actually related to uveitis.

Autoimmune Disorders

As I mentioned previously, autoimmune disorders are diseases that cause your immune system to attack parts of your body as if they were antigens. There are dozens of different types of autoimmune disorders, but let's talk about the ones that are mostly likely to occur simultaneously with uveitis and iritis:

Ankylosing Spondylitis

Ankylosing spondylitis is a form of arthritis that affects the spine. It most commonly affects men in their teens and twenties, but people of any age can get it. It causes the bones of the spine to fuse together resulting in extreme stiffness of the spine. The most common symptoms of ankylosing spondylitis are:

- Pain and stiffness in the lower back, buttocks, and hips. The pain often starts in the sacroiliac joints, where the spine meets the pelvic bone.

- Bony fusion is the word for overgrowth of bones, which is what causes back stiffness and other symptoms of ankylosing spondylitis. While the spine is the primary location, some people with this disease may experience fusing of the ribs to the spinal column or breastbone, a condition that can make taking deep breaths painful or impossible.

- Patients with ankylosing spondylitis may also experience inflammation of connective tissues such as ligaments and tendons.

- Because ankylosing spondylitis is a systemic disease, it can also cause other symptoms including fatigue, fever, inflammation of the eyes, and in serious cases, heart and lung problems.

At present, there is no cure for ankylosing spondylitis. Treatments can vary, but some of the most common treatments include non-steroidal anti-inflammatory medications (NSAIDS), steroidal injections, physical and occupational therapies, and anti-rheumatic drugs.

Sarcoidosis

Sarcoidosis is an autoimmune disorder that causes inflammation in various parts of the body, most commonly the lungs and lymph nodes. It is more common in women than in men, with the most frequent onset happening between the ages of 20 and 40. Sarcoidosis is more common amongst people of certain ethnicities. African Americans are between 10 and 17 times more likely to get sarcoidosis than Caucasians. Also, people of German, Irish, Puerto Rican or Scandinavian descent are at increased risk for the disease as well.

The most common symptoms of sarcoidosis are:

- Persistent dry cough
- Shortness of breath
- Fatigue

Other symptoms may include: reddish bumps on the skin, blurred vision, swollen joints, enlarged lymph glands, hoarse voice, pain in the hands and feet, kidney stones, enlarged liver, and heart arrhythmias.

There is no cure for sarcoidosis at present. Many patients who have it experience symptoms for a short time and they clear up on their own. For a few patients, however, sarcoidosis becomes a chronic condition. The treatment options are similar to those for uveitis, with the most common treatment being corticosteroids to help reduce inflammation and get rid of the cough that is commonly associated with sarcoidosis.

Crohn's Disease

Crohn's disease is an inflammatory disease of the bowels. It may be caused by a malfunction of the immune system, as other autoimmune diseases are. However, there are certain viruses and infections that appear to cause Crohn's disease as well. Because of that, it might be better classified as an inflammatory disease.

There is a hereditary component to Crohn's disease, and like sarcoidosis, people of certain ethnic heritages are more likely to get it than others. For example, people of Eastern European heritage, in particular, Ashkenazi Jews, are highly susceptible to Crohn's disease. Smoking cigarettes can also increase your chances of getting it.

The primary symptoms associated with Crohn's disease are stomach pains and frequent diarrhea. The diarrhea is sometimes bloody, and people with Crohn's disease may end up losing weight without trying as a result of diarrhea. Some of the less common symptoms include bowel blockages, *anal fissures* (tears in the tissue), *fistulas* (openings) between organs, and lesions or sores in the mouth.

There is no cure for Crohn's disease at the moment, but anti-inflammatory medications and careful diet control can help reduce or eliminate symptoms. A patient who has Crohn's disease but is asymptomatic is said to be in remission.

Rheumatoid Arthritis

Rheumatoid arthritis is an autoimmune disorder in which the body attacks connective tissues (ligaments and tendons) as though they were antigens. The primary symptoms are:

- Severe stiffness in the joints. While waking up with stiff joints is a common symptom of all types of arthritis, people with rheumatoid arthritis may take a long time (even several hours) for their joints to feel loose.

- Swelling in the joints. Fluid accumulates in the joints and causes them to become swollen and painful to touch.

- Joint pain. The swelling and inflammation of the joints cause the joints to become tender and sensitive to the touch. Over time, the inflammation can cause damage to the joints.

- Redness and warmth. The inflammation can cause the affected joints to redden and become warm to the touch.

Rheumatoid arthritis occurs most commonly in the hands, but any joint in the body can be affected including the hips, knees, elbows, jaw, and neck.

While the above symptoms are the most common, rheumatoid arthritis can also cause fatigue, sickness, decreased appetite, weight loss, and muscle aches – symptoms that some people with rheumatoid arthritis may mistake for the flu.

In serious cases, rheumatoid arthritis can cause the lungs or the lining around the heart to become inflamed. Most people with rheumatoid arthritis do not experience inflammation of the eyes, but for some people, uveitis is a side effect of rheumatoid arthritis.

There is no cure for rheumatoid arthritis, but early treatment can minimize damage to the joints and keep inflammation under control. The most common treatments include non-steroidal anti-inflammatory drugs (NSAIDs), disease-modifying antirheumatic drugs (DMARDs), steroids, and biologics (drugs that suppress the part of the immune system that is responsible for rheumatoid arthritis.)

Other Autoimmune Disorders

The above diseases are some of the most common autoimmune diseases linked to uveitis, but there are others. For example:

- Behcet's disease is a rare autoimmune disorder that causes inflammation of the blood vessels.

- Ulcerative colitis shares some similarities with Crohn's disease. It causes inflammation of the colon, including the development of lesions and sores.

- Kawasaki disease is a rare disease that occurs primarily in children. It causes inflammation of the blood vessels, including arteries, veins, and capillaries. In serious cases, it may cause heart damage.

- Lupus erythematosus is a systemic autoimmune disease that often starts with skin inflammation. When the disease becomes systemic, it can lead to inflammation of the internal organs.

Viral and Bacterial Infections

While autoimmune disorders are one of the most common causes of uveitis, bacterial and viral infections can cause the disease as well. Let's take a look at some of the most common culprits.

Human Immunodeficiency Virus (HIV)

You are probably familiar with HIV as the virus that causes AIDS (Acquired Immunodeficiency Syndrome). People who have HIV and AIDS tend to be susceptible to opportunistic infections – infections that would probably not affect people whose immune systems were operating at full capacity. Because HIV attacks the immune system directly, uveitis is a common problem for people who have the disease.

HIV is spread through direct sexual contact with an infected person or by sharing an intravenous needle with an infected person. When a person is first infected, the body's immune system tries to fight off the disease and the affected person may end up having flu-like symptoms that then disappear. However, the symptoms typically fade quickly and are unlikely to be linked to HIV unless the patient knows that he has been exposed. After that, the disease can be dormant for years.

Once the affected person's T-cell count drops below a certain level, HIV becomes AIDS. At that point the patient's immune system is damaged and deeply compromised. At this point, there is no cure for HIV and AIDS; but early intervention and drugs can help bolster the immune system and keep it from turning into AIDS.

Herpes Simplex Virus

Herpes is a sexually transmitted infection (STI) that can be spread through genital-to-genital, mouth-to-genital, or anus-to-genital contact. The most common symptom of herpes is the presence of lesions or sores on the affected areas. There are two basic forms of the virus: simplex one and simplex two. Simplex one is typically associated with oral herpes while simplex two is associated with genital herpes. However, either variation of the disease can appear anywhere on the body.

There is no cure for herpes, but people can and do manage the disease by taking anti-viral medications. The herpes virus lives in the nervous system, which may help explain why it can cause inflammation of the eyes.

Syphilis

Syphilis is a sexually transmitted bacterial infection that can be spread during unprotected sex. The most typical symptom of infection is the presence of a sore in the genital area. If it is left untreated, syphilis can spread to other areas of the body, causing rashes on the hands and feet. In serious cases, it can lead to systemic problems including heart disease.

Because syphilis is a bacterial infection, it can be easily cured with a high dose of penicillin or another antibiotic medication. People whose immune symptoms are already compromised in some way are more likely to catch syphilis than people whose immune systems are fully functional.

Tuberculosis

Like syphilis, tuberculosis is a bacterial infection that primarily affects the lungs, although it can affect other areas of the body too. It is spread when an infected person coughs, releasing aerosol droplets that contain the bacteria that cause the disease. Only a small amount of bacteria is required to spread the infection. People who are exposed to patients with tuberculosis are very likely to contract the disease unless they take precautions such as wearing protective gear.

Worldwide, the most common risk factor for tuberculosis is infection with HIV. A person with a healthy immune system could be exposed to tuberculosis bacteria and not get infected, but a person whose immune system is compromised is at much higher risk. While overall the number of tuberculosis cases has declined, it is still fairly common in developing countries where sanitation is poor, and HIV infection is widespread.

The typical treatment for tuberculosis is a high dose of an antibiotic medication such as penicillin or cyclosporin. In most people, antibiotics will clear up the infection. However, some people may end up having chronic tuberculosis.

While the diseases listed above are the most common viral and bacterial infections to cause uveitis, there are others. Here are a few to keep in mind:

- Toxoplasmosis is a bacterial infection that can pass from infected cats to humans. Infection in humans is rare but more common among people whose immune systems are compromised. It may also be spread from mother to child during birth.

- Cytomegalovirus is a virus that produces symptoms similar to those of mononucleosis. Again, it is rare except in patients whose immune systems are weakened or compromised.

- Varicella zoster virus is the virus that causes chickenpox in children and shingles in adults. There is a vaccine available, but again, people whose immune systems are compromised may be more likely to get shingles, which can then lead to uveitis.

- Lyme disease is a bacterial infection that is spread by infected ticks. It's a rare disease, but a serious one.

- Other bacterial infections that may cause or contribute to uveitis include brucellosis, leptospirosis, and toxocariasis.

Infections are less common as a cause of uveitis than autoimmune disorders, but it is still important to understand all of the causes so you can work with your doctor to identify other issues and treat them properly. A patient whose uveitis is caused by a bacterial infection may find that the uveitis clears up after taking antibiotics to treat the infection.

One of the most common theories about why uveitis is linked to these diseases and infections is that it is actually your body's way of dealing with eye infections. While it's clearly an overzealous response on the part of your immune system, the inflammation itself may be a sign that your body is fighting an intruder (or, in the case of autoimmune diseases, a perceived intruder).

For that reason, it can be helpful for people who have uveitis to make certain lifestyle changes in addition to taking medications to clear up the inflammation. While research into the causes of autoimmune diseases is ongoing, there is quite a bit of evidence to suggest that dietary changes can help. With that in mind, in the next chapter I'll talk about some of the foods that are most likely to cause or worsen inflammation, and why it might be worth eliminating them if you have chronic uveitis.

Chapter 7 – Uveitis and Diet

Now that we have discussed the link between autoimmune disorders and inflammation, it's time to talk about one of the things you can do to supplement the treatments your doctor gives you for uveitis.

You already know that uveitis is inflammation of the uvea. Inflammation is your body's natural response to infection, but that doesn't mean that infection is the only thing that can cause inflammation. Certain foods are known to cause inflammation, and eliminating them from your diet can help to reduce the pain and inflammation associated with uveitis.

Another dietary change to consider is increasing your consumption of foods that boost your immune system naturally. Because so many of the diseases that cause uveitis are caused by a weakened immune system, boosting your intake of foods containing antioxidants may help your body fight infection and keep it stronger in general. Let's start by talking about the foods that are most likely to cause inflammation.

Inflammatory Foods

Even if you haven't thought about it before, you probably know on some level that the foods you eat can sometimes cause inflammation. All of us have had times when we've eaten something that disagrees with us in some way, whether the result is an overzealous immune reaction like an allergic attack or a milder one like an upset stomach.

You're probably already familiar with some of the most common culprits because they have received a certain amount of media attention. For example, a significant percentage of the world's population is intolerant to lactose, the sugar found in dairy products. The prevalence of lactose-free milk is a testament to how widespread this particular food sensitivity is. The same goes for gluten, the protein found in wheat and other grains. Gluten-free foods are increasingly popular. In fact, gluten intolerance is specifically linked to Celiac disease, which is an autoimmune disorder.

While researchers are still investigating the link between diet and other autoimmune disorders such as rheumatoid arthritis, there is evidence to support the idea that eliminating inflammatory foods from your diet can help to decrease symptoms by reducing the amount of inflammation in the body. Here are some of the foods to consider eliminating:

- Gluten. As previously mentioned, gluten is the protein found in cultivated grains such as wheat, rye, and barley. It is also found in any foods made with these products, including flour, bread, pasta, couscous, and most baked goods. Eliminating gluten from your diet can be a challenge because it is so common, but there are many gluten-free products available now. Grains that do not contain gluten include rice, quinoa, amaranth, buckwheat, and millet. Legumes are also a good substitute because they are a great source of fiber.

- Dairy. Lactose intolerance is very common, affecting approximately 65% of the world's population. Lactose is a sugar that occurs naturally in dairy products such as milk, yogurt, and cheese. Lactose-free versions of many foods are available. You can also choose to substitute with dairy-free products such as almond milk, soy milk, coconut milk, or rice milk.

- Sugar. Sugar is a common culprit in inflammatory responses, and the typical North American diet contains far too much sugar to be healthy. Many manufactured and processed foods contain large amounts of added sugar. It is important to note that sugar can hide on food labels under a lot of different names. In general, avoid anything that ends in –ose, including dextrose, sucrose, maltose, lactose, galactose, and fructose. Other ingredients to look out for include high fructose corn syrup, corn sugar, molasses, and anything ending in –tol (maltitol, sorbitol, etc.)

- Artificial sweeteners. While sugar can cause inflammation, artificial sweeteners aren't much better for you. You will be better served by sweetening your food with raw honey or stevia (an all-natural sugar substitute) than you will be by using any of the following: saccharin, acesulfame, aspartame, sucralose, alitame, cyclamate, neohesperidine dihydrochalcone (NHDC), and advantame.

- Monosodium glutamate. Monosodium glutamate (MSG) is a common food additive and flavor enhancer that is used in many processed foods. Many of us are highly sensitive to it and can develop headaches and other inflammatory responses after eating it. It's also commonly used in Asian restaurants, but a good restaurant will allow you to order your food without MSG.

- Trans fats. Trans fat is a type of processed fat that has been linked to inflammation and other health issues, including heart disease. In general, any food that is naturally liquid at room temperature but has been processed into a solid as a trans fat. Examples include vegetable shortening and margarine, as well as any fat or oil listed on an ingredient label as *hydrogenated* or *partially hydrogenated*.

- Omega-6 fatty acids are not bad for you when they are eaten in the correct amounts. However, most people get far more Omega-6 than they need while not ingesting enough Omega-3, which helps to counteract the inflammatory effects of Omega-6. Omega-6 fatty acids are in many of the oils we use for cooking, including corn oil, soybean oil, peanut oil, grapeseed oil, cottonseed oil, sunflower oil, and safflower oil. Ideally, you should be getting equal amounts of Omega-6 and Omega-3. Most people, particularly in North America, get about 25 times as much Omega-6 as they do

Omega-3, which is why it's a major contributor to systemic inflammation.

- Nuts and seeds. For some people, particularly those who are sensitive to inflammation in the stomach and intestines, eliminating nuts and seeds from the diet can be helpful. The histamines in nuts can cause a strong immune response from the body that may lead to inflammation.

- Tomatoes and other nightshades. Fruits and vegetables in the nightshade family, including tomatoes, eggplants, peppers, and white potatoes, can cause inflammation in some people.

If you decide to try an anti-inflammatory diet, the best way to start is to eliminate all of the most common food culprits from your diet. If you notice an improvement in your symptoms, you can identify the foods that cause a problem by introducing them back into your diet one at a time. It's important only to add one thing at a time so you can pinpoint the foods that your body reacts to. If you try adding both gluten and nuts back to your diet at once, you'll have no way of knowing which one is responsible for the inflammation you experience.

Foods to Boost Immunity

Eliminating inflammatory foods is a good way to find out if your diet is exacerbating the symptoms of uveitis and any other diseases you may have, but it's not the only way that your diet can help improve your health. The other part of the equation is making sure to get the nutrients your body needs to fight off infection.

You're probably familiar with the term antioxidant, but even people who have heard of antioxidants might not be sure what the term means. Before we talk about the specific foods that can help to boost your immune system, let's talk about what antioxidants do. Their primary job is to protect your body from something called *oxidative stress*.

Oxidative stress is damage that is caused when the cells in your body are exposed to oxygen. If you have ever cut open an apple and watched it turn brown when it comes into contact with the air, you have seen oxidative stress in action.

What happens to your body when it experience oxidative stress is that your cells can lose electrons. When that occurs, the cell becomes something called a *free radical*. The cell is out of balance because of the missing electron, and it will do anything it can to regain an electron, including stealing one from a neighboring cell. The theft of an electron can set off a chain reaction, with each cell stealing an electron from the one next to it.

Antioxidants protect your body against this type of damage because they can loan an electron to a free radical, thus stopping the chain reaction in its tracks. Many of the foods we know as essential micronutrients (vitamins and minerals) have antioxidant properties. Here are some of the most common antioxidants along with a list of foods that contain them.

- Vitamin A is an essential micronutrient with powerful antioxidant properties. Vitamin A deficiencies have been linked directly to vision problems including macular degeneration. Many orange fruits and vegetables contain high amounts of Vitamin A, including sweet potatoes, carrots, mangos, papayas, butternut squash, peaches, and cantaloupe. Other good dietary sources of Vitamin A include dark leafy greens, fish, and liver.

- Vitamin C is another important vitamin that contains antioxidants. Most of us know that inadequate intake of Vitamin C can make it harder to fight off colds and viruses. Good dietary sources of Vitamin C include citrus fruits such as oranges, grapefruits, lemons, limes, and tangerines. Other good sources include dark leafy greens like spinach and kale, cruciferous vegetables like broccoli and

Brussels sprouts, and other fruits such as strawberries, pineapples, and raspberries.

- Vitamin E is great for your skin and hair, and it also has antioxidant properties to protect against inflammation. Good dietary sources of Vitamin E include avocados, almonds (if you're not sensitive to nuts), Swiss chard, spinach, and kale. Fatty fish such as salmon is also a good source of Vitamin E.

- Selenium is a mineral that has antioxidant properties. Some foods that are high in selenium include oysters, tuna, broccoli, Brazil nuts, pork, beef, lamb, poultry, and mushrooms.

- Lycopene is another powerful antioxidant that is particularly helpful for male reproductive health, among other things. Tomatoes and tomato products are excellent sources of lycopene. Other good dietary sources include watermelon, guava, and pink grapefruit.

- Lutein has antioxidant properties and is also a micronutrient that is particularly important for healthy eyesight. It has been shown to help reduce the risk of macular degeneration. Foods that contain large amounts of lutein include Brussels sprouts, peas, corn, beet greens, pumpkin, and asparagus.

Anti-Inflammatory Foods

In addition to eliminating foods that cause inflammation and adding antioxidants to your diet, there are also some specific foods that are particularly good at fighting inflammation. Here are some things to consider adding to your diet:

- Blueberries
- Coffee
- Dark chocolate
- Apples
- Olive oil

- Dark leafy greens

All of these foods include plant compounds called polyphenols, which have been shown to reduce inflammation.

Following an anti-inflammatory, immune-boosting diet won't cure uveitis, but it can help to reduce the symptoms and make flare-ups less severe. It might seem difficult to eliminate things like sugar from your diet, but the important thing is to weigh the difficulty against the painful reality of uveitis and how it impacts your life on a daily basis.

Chapter 8 – Iritis.org

One of the most challenging things about getting a diagnosis of uveitis or iritis – especially before the internet made it easier to find information about medical conditions – was that there was so little information available. I founded the Iritis Organization in 1994 shortly after I was diagnosed with uveitis. I wanted to provide detailed information and resources to other people who, like me, had been diagnosed with an unfamiliar and rare disease.

Today, the Iritis Organization is still relatively small. I run the website with help from a few volunteers who help me manage and moderate the forums. While the organization is small, the community on **Iritis.org** is large and growing every day. The forums have become a source of information and comfort for people who have uveitis.

I would like to invite you to visit the website. I have done my best to make it a place where you can find both information and support. Let me give you a quick overview of what you can expect to find there.

- Detailed information about iritis and uveitis, including an explanation of what the disease is, the most common symptoms, and what causes it.

- Links to another website, **Uveitis.org**, which has a comprehensive list of doctors who specialize in the treatment of uveitis and iritis. It is very important to see a specialist when you have uveitis. Your general practitioner may have heard of uveitis, but you need to see someone who is experienced in the diagnosis and management of the disease.

- Information regarding common treatments for uveitis and what they do. The treatment information includes discussion of common co-diagnoses and the complications that can arise if uveitis is not treated properly.

- I have a blog on the website that I use to explore topics related to uveitis and iritis. For example, I might talk about new research and medications to keep members updated as new information becomes available.

I hope to expand the site and make the information there more comprehensive in the future.

Support Community

The part of the site that I think is the most valuable to people who have been diagnosed with uveitis or iritis is the forum. When you have a disease that's rare and difficult to treat, as uveitis is, it is very important to have the ability to talk to other people who understand what it's like. Sharing experiences with people who truly understand them can be very healing.

What can you expect to find on the forum? Let me give you a taste of some of the main topics of discussion, as well as an overview of some of the specific sub forums you can find on the board:

- *Announcements.* This is a place where we post information and updates that may be helpful to the community. For example, we might post information about trials for a new uveitis drug, or a tutorial that shows you how to apply eye drops.

- *Introduce Yourself.* This is a special forum where new members can introduce themselves and talk about their specific experiences with uveitis. I started this particular area of the forum so that we could do a better job of keeping track of our members and the challenges they are facing. When you have a rare disease, it can be easy to feel as if you're all alone. A quick read through some of the posts in this forum will let you know that you're not.

- *Related Conditions.* In this area of the forum, members can talk about uveitis as it relates to other conditions they may have, including autoimmune disorders, viruses, and infections. You can share information with other members and get responses from our moderators that may help you get the treatment you need.

- *Additional Readings*. This is an informational area of the forum where you can read articles and papers related to the research and treatment of uveitis and iritis.

- *Iritis/Uveitis Specialists*. As anybody with a chronic disease can tell you, one of the keys to managing an illness successfully is having a good doctor. In this area of the forum, members talk about their experiences with specific doctors. If you're shopping for a new doctor, this is a great place to get an idea of what to expect. It can help you decide between two doctors, and most importantly, help you avoid doctors who aren't responsive.

- *Medical Information, Drugs, Etc.* This area of the forum is where we will share specific information related to the treatment of iritis and uveitis, including details about drugs and other potential treatments.

- *Parents' Forum.* This area of the website is specifically for parents whose children have received a diagnosis of iritis or uveitis. Dealing with a chronic disease in a child presents special challenges, and this is a place where you can share your story and get support from other parents whose children have uveitis.

The mission of the Iritis Organization is to offer support and valuable information to people who are battling acute and chronic uveitis. Having a chronic disease isn't easy. The recurring nature of uveitis – along with the fact that it can have such a significant impact on your quality of life – makes it a particularly challenging diagnosis to receive. When I was diagnosed, there wasn't much information available. It is still challenging to find information, but my goal is to make it easier by making my website a place where people can find the information and support they need.

Conclusion

Thank you for reading *Living with Uveitis*. I hope that you have found the information included in this book to be helpful. It can be extremely frustrating to get a diagnosis such as uveitis. It is natural for patients who are diagnosed to be hungry for information. The challenge for people with uveitis is that information is scarce.

One of the most frustrating things about uveitis is that, in so many cases, there is no explanation for how the patient caught the disease. To be told that you have a chronic disease with no cause and no cure is very difficult. The ironic thing about the stress and frustration that can occur as a result of a uveitis diagnosis is that stress can actually make inflammation worse. The last thing you want to do is to be feeling an emotion that exacerbates your condition, yet the lack of information about uveitis makes it difficult to avoid feelings of stress and anxiety.

There are a few important things I hope you take away from this book:

1. You're not alone. While uveitis is rare and many of the people in your life – including your doctor – may not have heard of it, there are other people out there who know how you feel. I understand, and so do the people who participate in the Iritis.org forum. Talking about your condition with people who understand what it's like and can empathize with your experiences is a big part of the healing process.

2. You're not helpless. While being told that there is no cure for uveitis is frustrating, that doesn't mean that there's nothing you can do. You can be a strong advocate for your own treatment. That includes learning as much as you can about the available treatments. The more you know, the better equipped you will be to talk to your doctor and make the best choices for your

own health and well-being.

3. Knowledge is power. One of the very best things you can do as a patient is to learn everything possible about your condition. Know what the latest research says, and find out what other people have experienced. Research your doctors and insist on getting the very best care available. The same goes for work, driving, and any other issue that's related to uveitis. When you know your rights and options, you can make the best possible choices.

4. It's not all about medicine. While corticosteroids and immunosuppressant drugs are an important part of controlling chronic uveitis, you can also take action by managing your diet. You may not be able to cure the disease, but you can certainly do things that will help reduce your symptoms and minimize flare-ups. Eliminating inflammatory foods, boosting your immune system, and eating

superfoods that help to reduce inflammation can make a big difference.

5. Support is key. Visiting the forums on my website, **iritis.org** is a great way to connect with other people who have uveitis and iritis. You deserve to have the best information possible. If your family and friends aren't supportive – or if they are, but they just don't understand what it's like to have uveitis – you can find dozens and dozens of people who do on our forums. No matter what you are experiencing, there is someone there who will understand exactly what it's like and who can offer support and warmth when you need it.

The other thing to remember is that you always have the right to ask questions and demand explanations from your health care providers. If you have a doctor who won't answer your questions, check out the area of our forum where members review specialists and find someone who is a better fit for you. You have a right to demand high-quality care. Many doctors don't understand uveitis. The best way to control the disease and ensure that you don't end up with complications is to find a uveitis specialist who will help you come up with a long-term plan to manage your symptoms and prevent flare-ups from occurring. If your current doctor isn't doing that, the best thing you can do is to find one who will.

I know how hard it can be to have uveitis. We depend on our eyes for more things than we realize. Having difficulty with your eyes can lead to practical problems, such as the inability to drive or perform your normal job duties. It can also cause emotional problems. Many people with uveitis feel cut off from their usual lives. The things they used to do to fill their time, such as reading, watching television or movies, or doing artistic work or practical things around the house, may be curtailed by the inflammation and pain associated with uveitis.

The good news is that there is more and more research being done to find a cure for uveitis. The more passionately the people who have uveitis advocate for a cure, the more likely it is that researchers will eventually find one.

In the meantime, I hope you will take advantage of the resources available at the **Iritis Organization**.

19776509R00070

Printed in Poland
by Amazon Fulfillment
Poland Sp. z o.o., Wrocław